A Beginner's Booklet on Acupuncture

A Beginner's Booklet on Acupuncture

Julia Chen

Better than Bonkers

Contents

First Printing, 2023

ISBN: 979-8-8690-2361-2
EISBN: 979-8-8690-3301-7

{ 1 }

What Is Acupuncture?

Introduction to Acupuncture: Unraveling the Tapestry of Healing

Acupuncture, a venerable alternative medical practice rooted in the ancient traditions of Chinese medicine, beckons with intrigue and captivation on a global scale. As we commence this enlightening journey into the realm of acupuncture, we extend a warm welcome to you, the curious seeker, to this beginners' guide. This art, often cloaked in mystery, holds the promise of unveiling therapeutic wonders. In this inaugural chapter, let's navigate through crucial points about acupuncture, laying the groundwork for a more profound exploration in the chapters that follow.

Historical Context: A Journey Through Time

Acupuncture's historical roots extend thousands of years, finding its genesis in ancient China and becoming an integral part of traditional Chinese medicine. Its enduring popularity and acceptance have transcended cultural boundaries, making significant inroads into the Western healthcare landscape.

Applications in Modern Healthcare: Bridging Ancient Wisdom and Contemporary Needs

Today, acupuncture stands as a widely embraced treatment, demonstrating efficacy in addressing a spectrum of ailments. From chronic issues like back pain and headaches to managing conditions such as osteoarthritis, alleviating postoperative discomfort, mitigating allergies, supporting cancer treatments, aiding stroke rehabilitation, and addressing infertility concerns, its applications are diverse. While sought as a less aggressive alternative, it's essential to note that acupuncture complements rather than replaces primary medical interventions.

Geographical Prevalence: A Global Tapestry of Healing

The practice of acupuncture has found its home in various corners of the world, with a notable presence in the United States, the United Kingdom, and Asia. Administered by skilled practitioners, acupuncture sessions are sought by those seeking holistic approaches to health and wellness.

The Mechanics of Acupuncture: Precision and Comfort

The term "acupuncture" derives from the Latin words "acus" (needle) and "punctura" (to puncture). The procedure involves the delicate insertion of fine needles into specific acupuncture points on the body. Needle sizes vary based on the targeted area, and patients are positioned comfortably as the needles gently penetrate the skin. Contrary to initial concerns, practitioners assure minimal discomfort, describing sensations akin to a subtle buzzing or stinging. Session durations vary, catering to the severity of health concerns.

Philosophical Underpinnings: Qi, Meridians, and Balance

At the heart of acupuncture lie principles from traditional Chinese medicine, where the human body is seen as an intricate network of energy pathways, or meridians, facilitating the circulation of Qi, a vital life force. This energy flow maintains balance, promoting overall health. Diseases, according to this philosophy, arise from imbalances in Qi flow due to external or internal factors.

Scientific Perspectives: Blending Ancient Wisdom with Contemporary Understanding

In the contemporary era, while concepts like Qi and meridians lack scientific proof, acupuncturists adopt alternative explanations. The prevailing theory centers on the body's biochemical response to needling, triggering the release of endorphins and adenosine, known for their pain-relieving and mood-enhancing properties. While acupuncture shows efficacy in relieving pain, scientific evidence supporting its broader effectiveness remains elusive.

Conclusion and Future Exploration: A Tapestry Unfolds

This initial exploration merely scratches the surface of acupuncture's multifaceted world. In the chapters ahead, we will delve into specific facets, unraveling intricacies, and exploring varied applications. Whether you're a newcomer or a seasoned explorer in acupuncture, deeper insights await. Are you prepared to embark on this enlightening expedition? Let's continue our exploration of acupuncture, a timeless art weaving its therapeutic tapestry across diverse cultures and healthcare landscapes.

{ 2 }

The History Of Acupuncture & How It Affects You

The Resilience of Chinese Medicine Through the Ages:

Long predating the advent of Western medicine, the Chinese civilization had already woven a rich tapestry of medical knowledge and healing practices. Across millennia, Chinese healers diligently honed and expanded their medicinal system, crafting intricate processes designed to channel the flow of energy within the human body, offering a formidable arsenal against various ailments.

A Journey Through Acupuncture's Origins:

In this preliminary chapter, we embark on an exploration of the genesis and evolution of acupuncture, tracing its roots from ancient China to its contemporary prominence and envisioning its role in the future of healthcare.

The Ancient Foundations:

While pinpointing the precise moment of acupuncture's inception remains elusive, its initial documentation emerges in the "Classic of Internal Medicine of the Yellow Emperor," a foundational text of Chinese medicine dating back to the 1st century BC. This ancient manuscript serves as the bedrock upon which the intricate techniques of acupuncture are built, providing enduring wisdom that resonates in the practices observed today.

The Ebb and Flow of Traditional Chinese Medicine:

With the advent of modern medicine on the global stage, traditional Chinese medicine, including acupuncture, encountered a period of skepticism and decline. The lack of a scientific basis rendered these practices seemingly outdated. Throughout the 20th century, the ascent of Western healthcare paradigms led to attempts to banish acupuncture and its traditional counterparts.

Resilience Amidst Turbulence:

In the face of these challenges, the National Medical Assembly's resolute rejection of calls to dismantle traditional

Chinese medicine in 1929 marked a pivotal moment. However, despite the resilience of these healing arts, they lingered in the shadows, overshadowed by the dominance of Western medical practices until the tumultuous period of the Long March in 1934.

The Long March: A Turning Point:

The Long March, a tumultuous era of political upheaval, provided an unexpected opening for traditional Chinese medicine, particularly acupuncture, to stage a comeback. As warfare ravaged the land, traditional Chinese doctors found a niche, employing acupuncture to save lives amidst the scarcity of conventional medical resources.

A Bridge Between East and West:

Though Western medicine remains skeptical of acupuncture's foundations in Qi and meridians, scholars have acknowledged its role in unraveling the intricacies of the human body's response to stimulation and stress. The Long March, in particular, served as a bridge, allowing traditional Chinese medicine, alongside Western practices, to coexist, providing patients with a spectrum of treatment options.

Acupuncture's Resurgence and Global Acceptance:

Following the establishment of the People's Republic of

China in 1948, a concerted effort to revive traditional Chinese medicine took root. By 1978, these practices, including acupuncture, found their way back into hospitals, fostering dedicated research departments committed to refining and enhancing these age-old healing methods.

Today's Landscape:

In the 21st century, the enduring legacy of traditional Chinese medicine, bolstered by its success in navigating the complexities of the modern age, has positioned acupuncture as a globally accepted and practiced form of medical treatment. Its roots, anchored in ancient wisdom, have weathered the tides of skepticism, paving the way for a harmonious integration of Eastern and Western medical philosophies. The intricate dance between tradition and innovation continues, ensuring that acupuncture remains a beacon of holistic healing across diverse corners of the world.

{ 3 }

The Concepts Of Qi & Meridians

Unraveling the Concepts Behind Acupuncture:

Before delving into the intricate world of acupuncture treatment, it is imperative to grasp the underlying concepts and terminology that constitute the foundation of this ancient healing art. Familiarizing yourself with these principles not only enhances your comprehension of the process but also prepares your mind and body for the journey that lies ahead.

Qi and its Role in Acupuncture:

At the core of acupuncture lies the belief in Qi, an essential energy that is thought to regulate the body's equilibrium and foster a connection with the universe. This vital force plays a pivotal role in maintaining natural balance, and acupuncture is seen as a means to influence and regulate the flow of Qi within the body.

Harmony in Traditional Chinese Medicine:

Traditional Chinese medicine aims to cultivate harmony within the body concerning both the major organs and the external environment. The interconnectedness of these elements is central to achieving optimal health and well-being.

The Foundation: Zang-Fu Organs, Qi, and Meridians:

In traditional Chinese medicine, the concept of Qi is intertwined with the zang-fu organs, meridians, and bodily substances like blood and plasma. These elements form the bedrock of life, allowing the organs and tissues to function harmoniously.

The term "zang-fu" collectively refers to the twelve major organs, with the first six being the zang organs (heart, lungs, kidney, liver, spleen, and pericardium) and the remaining six termed as the fu organs (stomach, gallbladder, small and large intestine, bladder, and the unique san jiao). Each zang organ is complemented by a specific fu organ, and any imbalance between them can disrupt the flow of Qi, potentially leading to illness.

The Circulation of Qi Through Meridians:

Qi circulates through the body via pathways known as meridians. These channels ensure the regular flow of Qi through the organs and tissues, promoting health and preventing illness. Disruptions, such as accumulations of Qi in specific areas, can result in blockages that disturb the delicate balance of the entire body.

The Meridian Connection:

The intricate network of meridians establishes a connection between each vital organ and its corresponding pathway for Qi flow. There are twelve primary meridians, each paired with a zang-fu organ. These pairings include Lungs & Large Intestine, Stomach & Spleen, Heart & Small Intestine, Bladder & Kidneys, Liver & Gall Bladder, and Pericardium and San Jiao. These meridians not only flow throughout the body but also form connections with each zang-fu organ pair.

Enduring Concepts in Contemporary Healing:

Despite the passage of thousands of years, the concepts of Qi, zang-fu organs, and meridians continue to play a pivotal role in various branches of Chinese healing. Regardless of scientific validation, these principles offer a profound understanding of how treatments, including acupuncture, operate. Armed with this knowledge, individuals can make informed decisions about their health and explore treatments that resonate with their holistic well-being.

{ 4 }

Is Acupuncture Safe & Is It Right For Me?

Informed Decision-Making in Acupuncture:

Just like any medical treatment, the choice to undergo acupuncture warrants careful consideration. Patients are advised to embark on this journey with a well-informed mindset, understanding both the potential benefits and drawbacks, as well as the conceivable health risks and side effects associated with the procedure.

Understanding Suitability and Safety:

For those exploring traditional Chinese medicine, particularly considering acupuncture as a form of treatment, consulting with a healthcare provider becomes a crucial prerequisite. While acupuncture is generally deemed safe due to its non-invasive and painless nature, determining if one is a suitable candidate involves a thorough evaluation of individual health conditions. It is essential to inquire whether certain health concerns or pre-existing conditions might interact with or contraindicate acupuncture.

Acupuncture's Fundamental Goal:

To revisit the essence of acupuncture, it is an integral facet of traditional Chinese medicine, seamlessly integrated into mainstream medical practices today. The primary objective of acupuncture is to stimulate the body's major acupoints, facilitating the proper regulation of Qi or vital energy distribution. These acupoints are intricately linked to the 12 major organs known as zang-fu organs in traditional Chinese medicine, highlighting the interconnectedness between acupuncture and the body's overall balance and health.

Considerations Before Treatment:

Before embarking on acupuncture, individuals must acquaint themselves with the intricacies of the procedure. Acknowledging that acupuncture involves the insertion of very fine, pre-sterilized needles is essential. If an individual possesses a low pain tolerance or harbors a fear of needles, it may not be the most suitable mode of treatment. Fortunately, alternative forms of medicine exist, providing viable options for those with specific preferences or concerns.

Ideal Candidates for Acupuncture:

Acupuncture has been acclaimed for its potential to address a myriad of health concerns, ranging from common ailments to more severe conditions. It has demonstrated efficacy in issues such as infertility, obesity, headaches, and muscle pain, with anecdotal evidence supporting its role in alleviating chemotherapy side effects like nausea and vomiting. However, it is essential to manage expectations, as acupuncture is not a quick fix but a therapeutic journey that requires time, commitment, and regular recalibration.

Improving General Health and Well-being:

Many individuals turn to acupuncture to enhance their overall health. The treatment, known for its harmonizing effect on the body, is particularly beneficial for those seeking to improve their well-being and energy levels.

Addressing Fertility Issues:

Acupuncture is often recommended for individuals grappling with fertility challenges. For men, it may contribute to increased sperm production. Women, on the other hand, may find acupuncture helpful in regulating menstruation and correcting hormonal imbalances contributing to conditions like PCOS and other menstrual issues.

Relief for Fatigue and Chronic Pain:

Individuals experiencing chronic fatigue or persistent pain in various body parts can also benefit from acupuncture. The treatment is known to offer relief by addressing imbalances in the body's energy flow, providing a holistic approach to managing fatigue and discomfort.

In essence, before embracing acupuncture as a form of treatment, individuals are encouraged to delve into the specifics of their health, preferences, and treatment goals. Armed with this understanding, they can make informed decisions that align with their unique needs and contribute to their overall well-being.

Conditions That Can Be Treated With Acupuncture

A Comprehensive Exploration of Acupuncture's Therapeutic Impact:

Holistic Philosophy:

Acupuncture, deeply rooted in traditional Chinese medicine, embodies a holistic philosophy that goes beyond merely treating symptoms. It approaches the body as an interconnected system where the flow of vital energy, or Qi, plays a pivotal role in maintaining health and preventing illness. This holistic perspective involves meticulous attention to the body as a whole, major organs, and the dynamic interplay of energies that sustain life.

The Orchestrated Dance of Qi and Major Organs:

At the heart of acupuncture lies the nuanced interaction

with the 12 major organs as identified in Chinese medicine. Rather than just alleviating specific symptoms, acupuncture seeks to optimize the functioning of these organs, fostering an environment of balance and harmony. The precise stimulation of acupoints facilitates a cascade of effects, encouraging overall health and rectifying imbalances that may lead to various ailments.

Targeted Relief for Ailments:

Acupuncture's therapeutic range extends from the commonplace to the intricate, offering targeted relief for various conditions:

1. Headaches:

    Acupuncture has proven efficacy in providing relief for headaches, particularly migraines. The application of electroacupuncture in 20 sessions over a month has been shown to significantly reduce the frequency of migraines, offering tangible relief.

2. Seasonal Allergies:

    For those grappling with seasonal allergies resistant to conventional antihistamines, acupuncture emerges as a viable alternative. A series of at least 12 sessions may not only alleviate symptoms but also reduce the dependence on medication.

3. Mood Swings or Imbalances:

    Beyond the physical realm, acupuncture's positive influence extends to emotional well-being. Over a span of three months, it has demonstrated its capacity to treat depression by stimulating channels responsible for regulating endorphin production, contributing to an improved mood.

4. Acid Reflux and Heartburn:

Addressing digestive concerns, acupuncture aids in the regulation of acid secretion. A month-long course of regular sessions can provide a soothing alternative for those dealing with acid reflux and heartburn, eliminating the need for pharmaceutical intervention.

5. Heart Problems:

As a complement to a healthy lifestyle, acupuncture stands out for its ability to alleviate stress, lower cholesterol levels, and regulate blood pressure. This holistic approach contributes to the overall well-being of the cardiovascular system.

6. Sleep Disorders:

By stimulating acupoints, acupuncture induces the release of chemicals that facilitate the body's relaxation process. The resulting increase in neurotransmitters offers relief from insomnia and other sleep-related issues, promoting a more restful sleep.

World Health Organization (WHO) Recognition:

The World Health Organization (WHO) has conducted controlled clinical trials, recognizing acupuncture's efficacy in treating a diverse array of conditions. This endorsement includes relief from muscular spasms, joint pain, sciatica, dental pain, nausea, vomiting, postoperative pain, stroke, hypertension, depression, and complications related to childbirth. Additionally, acupuncture has shown promise in addressing menstrual and fertility problems for women.

A Complementary Approach to Well-being:

While acupuncture unquestionably stands as a valuable supportive treatment, it is crucial to view it as a complementary approach rather than a standalone remedy. Patients are advised to integrate acupuncture into a comprehensive healthcare strategy, recognizing its potential for temporary relief and enhancement of overall well-being. In doing so, individuals can unlock the full spectrum of benefits that acupuncture offers on their journey toward health and vitality.

{ **6** }

Acupuncture Techniques

Delving Deeper into Acupuncture Techniques:

As we unravel the intricacies of acupuncture, it becomes apparent that this ancient healing art is not just about needles but involves a nuanced set of techniques and approaches. Acupuncture, in its essence, utilizes pre-sterilized fine needles to stimulate the body's primary acupuncture points, employing methods that are both delicate and sophisticated.

Painless Precision with Fine Needles:

The very thought of needles may evoke apprehension, but the reality of acupuncture is far from intimidating. The needles used are delicately crafted, often slightly thicker than human hair. Their thickness and size vary based on the targeted area, with the most common type having a length of approximately 1.5 inches. The entire process is meticulously designed to ensure a painless experience for the patient.

Nuances of Needle Insertion:

Acupuncture practitioners are adept at employing various techniques for needle insertion, tailored to the specific requirements of each acupoint. Traditional practices involve inserting needles at an angle of 15 degrees or more, sometimes with the skin surface gently stretched to facilitate the needle's entry. A guide tube may also be utilized, ensuring precise placement without discomfort. As the needle is smoothly inserted, patients may experience sensations such as heaviness, tingling, or electrical pulses, collectively known as "de qi" or "the arrival of qi." This sensation, although varying among patients, is rarely associated with extreme pain, its intensity influenced by both health conditions and acupoint locations.

Beyond Needle Insertion:

While needle insertion remains the cornerstone of acupuncture, various techniques expand the realm of this ancient practice. These techniques, often chosen based on the specific ailment and patient comfort, include:

1. Acupressure:

A needle-free technique where acupoints are stimulated using hands and fingers, akin to a massage. Ideal for those with a low pain threshold, acupressure is effective in alleviating muscle pain and promoting the overall flow of Qi in the body.

2. *Moxibustion and Cupping:*

Widely popular and often integrated into massage parlors and spas, these techniques introduce heat to stimulate acupuncture points. Moxibustion utilizes heated needles, while cupping employs small glass cups to enhance Qi flow in specific body areas. These techniques are particularly beneficial for relieving muscle pain, spasms, and aiding in the elimination of body waste.

In essence, acupuncture transcends the simplicity of needle insertion, embracing a spectrum of techniques designed to cater to diverse patient needs and health conditions. This multifaceted approach underscores the adaptability and richness inherent in the practice of acupuncture, making it a truly holistic and personalized form of healing.

{ 7 }

Things To Consider Before Getting Treatment

Navigating the Journey of Acupuncture: A Holistic Approach to Health

The effectiveness of acupuncture, akin to diverse medical treatments, varies individually. Consulting a physician and conducting thorough research is paramount before committing to any medical treatment, irrespective of the health condition. Acupuncture, a cornerstone of traditional Chinese medicine, is widely embraced for its myriad health benefits. Despite rare reports of adverse effects, a thorough consideration of pros and cons is crucial.

Understanding the Gradual Transformation:

Acupuncture, promising comprehensive well-being, necessitates a realistic mindset. Unlike quick fixes such as surgery or medications, acupuncture requires commitment beyond a few sessions for optimal results. The frequency of sessions is contingent upon the severity and nature of the condition being treated. Prepare for bodily changes as acupuncture harmonizes the body's equilibrium, leading to sensations like fatigue, light-headedness, or emotional releases – indicative of the positive "de qi" or the arrival of Qi.

Navigating Sensations and Side Effects:

Embrace sensations and side effects as integral components of the acupuncture journey. Sensations like fatigue, light-headedness, or emotional outbursts signify the recalibration of Qi. Address unusual side effects or persistent pain promptly by consulting your acupuncturist. As Qi achieves balance, seize the opportunity to instigate broader health changes. Regular sessions enhance holistic well-being, making it essential to mentally prepare for purging negativity contributing to Qi imbalances and eventual illnesses.

Overcoming Doubts and Seeking Expert Guidance:

Doubts about pursuing acupuncture are natural, underscoring the importance of considering the aforementioned points. Acknowledge that treatment outcomes vary among individuals. To ensure you're in capable hands, consult an expert and licensed acupuncturist. While guarantees are elusive in healthcare, expert guidance minimizes uncertainties, fostering confidence in the transformative potential of acupuncture.

The Post-Acupuncture Landscape:

Post-acupuncture, recognize it as a pivotal chapter in your health improvement journey. Multiple sessions are imperative for lasting results, and the post-treatment phase demands adherence to specific guidelines. Side effects such as dizziness, headaches, fatigue, or emotional shifts, though common, typically signify positive Qi flow adjustments.

Acknowledging the Holistic Benefits:

Acupuncture is not just a treatment; it's a holistic approach that encourages individuals to embark on a transformative journey. By understanding its gradual impact, addressing sensations and side effects, and embracing broader lifestyle changes, individuals can harness the full potential of acupuncture. As Tim Daly rightly notes, "Thank God for Acupuncture, it's been around for 2000 years. It's not going anyplace, and people use it all of the time for a variety of cures and to avoid illnesses." The journey of acupuncture is an ongoing commitment to holistic well-being and the pursuit of a balanced, healthier life.

{ 8 }

After Treatment...Now What?

Post-Acupuncture Guidance: Nurturing the Effects of Healing

You've embraced acupuncture to address your ailment, completing the session in the clinic. This marks a significant chapter in your health journey. While lasting results aren't immediate, a series of sessions enhances the benefits. Post-acupuncture, follow crucial guidelines to maximize the positive effects and understand common side effects.

Immediate Post-Treatment Care:

Consider the post-acupuncture period as essential for health improvement. Relaxation is paramount, requiring a few hours of downtime to allow your refreshed system to absorb the session's effects. Avoid strenuous activities that induce stress and opt for light exercises like walking or yoga during the recovery period. If you experience discomfort or tingling, applying heat contributes to relaxation, alleviating residual sensations.

Understanding Normal Side Effects:

Post-acupuncture, normal side effects like dizziness, head-aches, tiredness, and heightened emotions are considered positive. These signify an improvement in Qi flow within your body, part of the holistic benefits of acupuncture. It's crucial to recognize these effects as indicators of the treatment's positive impact.

Addressing Soreness and Fatigue:

Soreness and fatigue are common after acupuncture, reflecting the body's recalibration. To preserve the positive effects, it's advisable to take it easy, avoiding strain. If soreness occurs in areas untouched by needles, consult your acupuncturist or healthcare provider promptly, as it may signal underlying issues needing attention. Fatigue indicates the treatment's effectiveness; rest immediately after and refrain from driving.

Navigating Emotional Changes:

Acupuncture may trigger emotional outbursts or mood swings as negative emotions are released. Embrace this as a positive aspect contributing to both physical and emotional well-being. Continued sessions will support overall improvement, making emotional health an integral part of the transformative journey.

Celebrating the Culmination:

Congratulations on reaching the pinnacle of the acupuncture guide. Needles, as tools for adjusting bodily functions, embody the principle behind acupuncture. Both ancient Chinese and modern Western practitioners have harnessed this technique for chronic disease relief, emphasizing its safety and positive impact.

Understanding Acupuncture Practices:

There are two overarching acupuncture practices today: Traditional Chinese Medicine (TCM) and medical acupuncture. TCM relies on the concept of Qi and meridians, using longer needles inserted deeper into acupuncture points. Medical acupuncture, practiced by Western medical school graduates, utilizes shorter, shallower insertions based on anatomical data. The choice between TCM and medical acupuncture is personal, balancing philosophies and comfort levels.

Conditions Treated by Acupuncture:

A broad spectrum of ailments, from asthma to anxiety, finds treatment in acupuncture. While TCM practitioners view health conditions as Qi flow imbalances, Western acupuncturists often focus on pain control. Extensive research supports acupuncture's efficacy in conditions like migraines, arthritis, and neuralgias, primarily through the gate-control theory of pain.

Expected Results and Puncture Session Outcome:

It's crucial to recognize that acupuncture complements existing medical therapy. Patient adherence to prescribed medication is paramount. A course of acupuncture, lasting weeks to months, varies based on the medical condition's complexity. Results begin manifesting after several sessions, with some conditions temporarily worsening before improvement.

Embracing Acupuncture's Legacy:

Acupuncture, a timeless gift from ancient sages, stands as a widely accepted practice in modern medicine. Its effectiveness, reproducibility, and safety offer relief to millions. As Tim Daly aptly states, "Thank God for Acupuncture, it's been around for 2000 years. It's not going anyplace, and people use it all of the time for a variety of cures and to avoid illnesses." The journey of acupuncture is an enduring commitment to holistic well-being, embracing the wisdom of ancient healing practices in our contemporary world.